This notebook belongs to:

____

Published by: Character Designs

Blood Sugar Tracker

Date	M	Blood Sugar			Food(s) Eaten Before Testing
		Fasting	1 Hour	2 Hours	

Blood Sugar Tracker

Date	M	Blood Sugar			Food(s) Eaten Before Testing
		Fasting	1 Hour	2 Hours	

Blood Sugar Tracker

Date	M	Blood Sugar			Food(s) Eaten Before Testing
		Fasting	1 Hour	2 Hours	

Blood Sugar Tracker

Date	M	Blood Sugar			Food(s) Eaten Before Testing
		Fasting	1 Hour	2 Hours	

Blood Sugar Tracker

Date	M	Blood Sugar			Food(s) Eaten Before Testing
		Fasting	1 Hour	2 Hours	

Blood Sugar Tracker

Date	M	Blood Sugar			Food(s) Eaten Before Testing
		Fasting	1 Hour	2 Hours	

Blood Sugar Tracker

Date	M	Blood Sugar			Food(s) Eaten Before Testing
		Fasting	1 Hour	2 Hours	

Blood Sugar Tracker

Date	M	Blood Sugar			Food(s) Eaten Before Testing
		Fasting	1 Hour	2 Hours	

Blood Sugar Tracker

Date	M	Blood Sugar			Food(s) Eaten Before Testing
		Fasting	1 Hour	2 Hours	

Blood Sugar Tracker

Date	M	Blood Sugar			Food(s) Eaten Before Testing
		Fasting	1 Hour	2 Hours	

Blood Sugar Tracker

Date	M	Blood Sugar			Food(s) Eaten Before Testing
		Fasting	1 Hour	2 Hours	

Blood Sugar Tracker

Date	M	Blood Sugar			Food(s) Eaten Before Testing
		Fasting	1 Hour	2 Hours	

Blood Sugar Tracker

Date	M	Blood Sugar			Food(s) Eaten Before Testing
		Fasting	1 Hour	2 Hours	

Blood Sugar Tracker

Date	M	Blood Sugar			Food(s) Eaten Before Testing
		Fasting	1 Hour	2 Hours	

Blood Sugar Tracker

Date	M	Blood Sugar			Food(s) Eaten Before Testing
		Fasting	1 Hour	2 Hours	

Blood Sugar Tracker

Date	M	Blood Sugar			Food(s) Eaten Before Testing
		Fasting	1 Hour	2 Hours	

Blood Sugar Tracker

Date	M	Blood Sugar			Food(s) Eaten Before Testing
		Fasting	1 Hour	2 Hours	

Blood Sugar Tracker

Date	M	Blood Sugar			Food(s) Eaten Before Testing
		Fasting	1 Hour	2 Hours	

Blood Sugar Tracker

Date	M	Blood Sugar			Food(s) Eaten Before Testing
		Fasting	1 Hour	2 Hours	

Blood Sugar Tracker

Date	M	Blood Sugar			Food(s) Eaten Before Testing
		Fasting	1 Hour	2 Hours	

Blood Sugar Tracker

Date	M	Blood Sugar			Food(s) Eaten Before Testing
		Fasting	1 Hour	2 Hours	

Blood Sugar Tracker

Date	M	Blood Sugar			Food(s) Eaten Before Testing
		Fasting	1 Hour	2 Hours	

Blood Sugar Tracker

Date	M	Blood Sugar			Food(s) Eaten Before Testing
		Fasting	1 Hour	2 Hours	

Blood Sugar Tracker

Date	M	Blood Sugar			Food(s) Eaten Before Testing
		Fasting	1 Hour	2 Hours	

Blood Sugar Tracker

Date	M	Blood Sugar			Food(s) Eaten Before Testing
		Fasting	1 Hour	2 Hours	

Blood Sugar Tracker

Date	M	Blood Sugar			Food(s) Eaten Before Testing
		Fasting	1 Hour	2 Hours	

Blood Sugar Tracker

Date	M	Blood Sugar			Food(s) Eaten Before Testing
		Fasting	1 Hour	2 Hours	

Blood Sugar Tracker

Date	M	Blood Sugar			Food(s) Eaten Before Testing
		Fasting	1 Hour	2 Hours	

Blood Sugar Tracker

Date	M	Blood Sugar			Food(s) Eaten Before Testing
		Fasting	1 Hour	2 Hours	

Blood Sugar Tracker

Date	M	Blood Sugar			Food(s) Eaten Before Testing
		Fasting	1 Hour	2 Hours	

Blood Sugar Tracker

Date	M	Blood Sugar			Food(s) Eaten Before Testing
		Fasting	1 Hour	2 Hours	

Blood Sugar Tracker

Date	M	Blood Sugar			Food(s) Eaten Before Testing
		Fasting	1 Hour	2 Hours	

Blood Sugar Tracker

Date	M	Blood Sugar			Food(s) Eaten Before Testing
		Fasting	1 Hour	2 Hours	

Blood Sugar Tracker

Date	M	Blood Sugar			Food(s) Eaten Before Testing
		Fasting	1 Hour	2 Hours	

Blood Sugar Tracker

Date	M	Blood Sugar			Food(s) Eaten Before Testing
		Fasting	1 Hour	2 Hours	

Blood Sugar Tracker

Date	M	Blood Sugar			Food(s) Eaten Before Testing
		Fasting	1 Hour	2 Hours	

Blood Sugar Tracker

Date	M	Blood Sugar			Food(s) Eaten Before Testing
		Fasting	1 Hour	2 Hours	

Blood Sugar Tracker

Date	M	Blood Sugar			Food(s) Eaten Before Testing
		Fasting	1 Hour	2 Hours	

Blood Sugar Tracker

Date	M	Blood Sugar			Food(s) Eaten Before Testing
		Fasting	1 Hour	2 Hours	

Blood Sugar Tracker

Date	M	Blood Sugar			Food(s) Eaten Before Testing
		Fasting	1 Hour	2 Hours	

Blood Sugar Tracker

Date	M	Blood Sugar			Food(s) Eaten Before Testing
		Fasting	1 Hour	2 Hours	

Blood Sugar Tracker

Date	M	Blood Sugar			Food(s) Eaten Before Testing
		Fasting	1 Hour	2 Hours	

Blood Sugar Tracker

Date	M	Blood Sugar			Food(s) Eaten Before Testing
		Fasting	1 Hour	2 Hours	

Blood Sugar Tracker

Date	M	Blood Sugar			Food(s) Eaten Before Testing
		Fasting	1 Hour	2 Hours	

Blood Sugar Tracker

Date	M	Blood Sugar			Food(s) Eaten Before Testing
		Fasting	1 Hour	2 Hours	

Blood Sugar Tracker

Date	M	Blood Sugar			Food(s) Eaten Before Testing
		Fasting	1 Hour	2 Hours	

Blood Sugar Tracker

Date	M	Blood Sugar			Food(s) Eaten Before Testing
		Fasting	1 Hour	2 Hours	

Blood Sugar Tracker

Date	M	Blood Sugar			Food(s) Eaten Before Testing
		Fasting	1 Hour	2 Hours	

Blood Sugar Tracker

Date	M	Blood Sugar			Food(s) Eaten Before Testing
		Fasting	1 Hour	2 Hours	

Blood Sugar Tracker

Date	M	Blood Sugar			Food(s) Eaten Before Testing
		Fasting	1 Hour	2 Hours	

Blood Sugar Tracker

Date	M	Blood Sugar			Food(s) Eaten Before Testing
		Fasting	1 Hour	2 Hours	

Blood Sugar Tracker

Date	M	Blood Sugar			Food(s) Eaten Before Testing
		Fasting	1 Hour	2 Hours	

Blood Sugar Tracker

Date	M	Blood Sugar			Food(s) Eaten Before Testing
		Fasting	1 Hour	2 Hours	

Blood Sugar Tracker

Date	M	Blood Sugar			Food(s) Eaten Before Testing
		Fasting	1 Hour	2 Hours	

Blood Sugar Tracker

Date	M	Blood Sugar			Food(s) Eaten Before Testing
		Fasting	1 Hour	2 Hours	

Blood Sugar Tracker

Date	M	Blood Sugar			Food(s) Eaten Before Testing
		Fasting	1 Hour	2 Hours	

Blood Sugar Tracker

Date	M	Blood Sugar			Food(s) Eaten Before Testing
		Fasting	1 Hour	2 Hours	

Blood Sugar Tracker

Date	M	Blood Sugar			Food(s) Eaten Before Testing
		Fasting	1 Hour	2 Hours	

Blood Sugar Tracker

Date	M	Blood Sugar			Food(s) Eaten Before Testing
		Fasting	1 Hour	2 Hours	

Blood Sugar Tracker

Date	M	Blood Sugar			Food(s) Eaten Before Testing
		Fasting	1 Hour	2 Hours	

Blood Sugar Tracker

Date	M	Blood Sugar			Food(s) Eaten Before Testing
		Fasting	1 Hour	2 Hours	

Blood Sugar Tracker

Date	M	Blood Sugar			Food(s) Eaten Before Testing
		Fasting	1 Hour	2 Hours	

Blood Sugar Tracker

Date	M	Blood Sugar			Food(s) Eaten Before Testing
		Fasting	1 Hour	2 Hours	

Blood Sugar Tracker

Date	M	Blood Sugar			Food(s) Eaten Before Testing
		Fasting	1 Hour	2 Hours	

Blood Sugar Tracker

Date	M	Blood Sugar			Food(s) Eaten Before Testing
		Fasting	1 Hour	2 Hours	

Blood Sugar Tracker

Date	M	Blood Sugar			Food(s) Eaten Before Testing
		Fasting	1 Hour	2 Hours	

Blood Sugar Tracker

Date	M	Blood Sugar			Food(s) Eaten Before Testing
		Fasting	1 Hour	2 Hours	

Blood Sugar Tracker

Date	M	Blood Sugar			Food(s) Eaten Before Testing
		Fasting	1 Hour	2 Hours	

Blood Sugar Tracker

Date	M	Blood Sugar			Food(s) Eaten Before Testing
		Fasting	1 Hour	2 Hours	

Blood Sugar Tracker

Date	M	Blood Sugar			Food(s) Eaten Before Testing
		Fasting	1 Hour	2 Hours	

Blood Sugar Tracker

Date	M	Blood Sugar			Food(s) Eaten Before Testing
		Fasting	1 Hour	2 Hours	

Blood Sugar Tracker

Date	M	Blood Sugar			Food(s) Eaten Before Testing
		Fasting	1 Hour	2 Hours	

Blood Sugar Tracker

Date	M	Blood Sugar			Food(s) Eaten Before Testing
		Fasting	1 Hour	2 Hours	

Blood Sugar Tracker

Date	M	Blood Sugar			Food(s) Eaten Before Testing
		Fasting	1 Hour	2 Hours	

Blood Sugar Tracker

Date	M	Blood Sugar			Food(s) Eaten Before Testing
		Fasting	1 Hour	2 Hours	

Blood Sugar Tracker

Date	M	Blood Sugar			Food(s) Eaten Before Testing
		Fasting	1 Hour	2 Hours	

Blood Sugar Tracker

Date	M	Blood Sugar			Food(s) Eaten Before Testing
		Fasting	1 Hour	2 Hours	

Blood Sugar Tracker

Date	M	Blood Sugar			Food(s) Eaten Before Testing
		Fasting	1 Hour	2 Hours	

Blood Sugar Tracker

Date	M	Blood Sugar			Food(s) Eaten Before Testing
		Fasting	1 Hour	2 Hours	

Blood Sugar Tracker

Date	M	Blood Sugar			Food(s) Eaten Before Testing
		Fasting	1 Hour	2 Hours	

Takeaway notes:

____

____

____

____

____

Year of use:

____